ULCERATIVE COLITIS COOKBOOK For Seniors

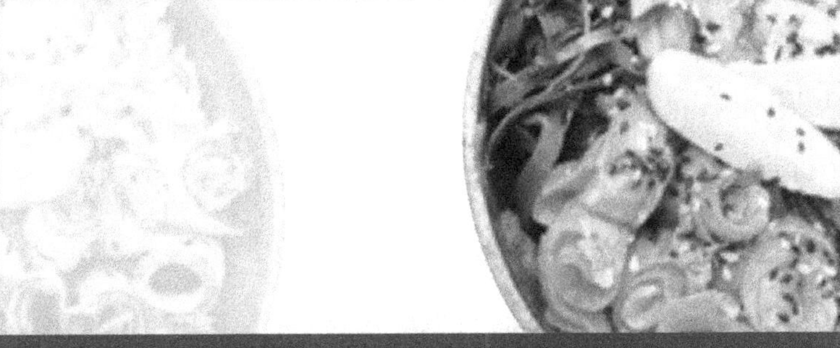

Delicious And Healthy Dairy Free, Low Fiber Recipes To Relieve The Symptoms And Complications In Colitis Patients

LEONA BUTLER

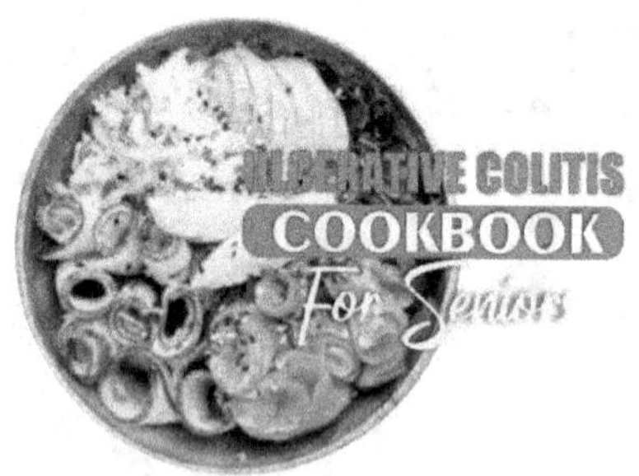
ULCERATIVE COLITIS
COOKBOOK
For Seniors

Table Of Content

2. Baked salmon with quinoa and roasted zucchini.

3. Turkey and vegetable stir-fry with brown rice.

4. Spinach and feta omelette with a side of roasted bell peppers.

5. Lentil soup with whole-grain toast.

6. Grilled shrimp salad with mixed greens and a light vinaigrette.

7. Baked cod with sautéed spinach and quinoa.

8. Turkey and vegetable wrap with a gluten-free tortilla.

9. Mashed butternut squash with roasted chicken breast.

10. Quinoa and roasted vegetable bowl with a touch of olive oil.

CHAPTER 5

DINNER RECIPES

1. Baked Salmon with Quinoa and Steamed Vegetables

2. Mashed Sweet Potatoes with Grilled Chicken and Green Beans:

3. Turkey and Vegetable Stir-Fry with Brown Rice:

4. Grilled Tilapia with Lemon Herb Quinoa and Roasted Zucchini Grilled Tilapia with Lemon Herb

5. Chicken and Rice Soup with Carrots and Spinach

6. Baked Cod with Cilantro Lime Rice and Steamed Asparagus gus:

7. Quinoa Salad with Grilled Shrimp, Cherry Tomatoes, and Avocado

8. Spinach and Feta Stuffed Chicken Breast with Mashed Cauliflower

9. Vegetable and Lentil Stew with Whole Grain Bread

10. Roasted Turkey Breast with Butternut Squash Mash and Sauteed Kale

BONUS

The Paperback Of This Version Has A Free 14 Weeks Meal Planner
_Toc157213432

30 DAY MEAL PLAN

CONCLUSION

Abstract

This novel Ulcerative Colitis Cookbook for Seniors addresses the specific dietary requirements of older people living with this chronic inflammatory disorder. The cookbook, designed to improve both nutritional intake and culinary delight, contains a varied selection of delectable and readily digested recipes.

Nutritionists have expertly developed the meals, which prioritize foods known to reduce inflammation, enhance intestinal health, and ensure optimal nutrient absorption. With a focus on simplicity, the cookbook caters to a wide range of cooking abilities, making it accessible to seniors with various culinary capabilities.

Each meal has been deliberately crafted to supply necessary nutrients while also accommodating dietary restrictions common to ulcerative colitis patients. Beyond recipes, the cookbook provides seniors with practical ideas for meal planning, grocery shopping, and eating a balanced diet, allowing them to take charge of their health through fun and fulfilling meals.

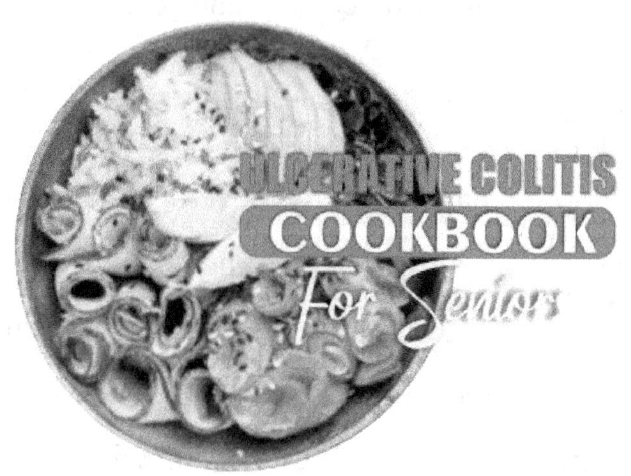

Introduction

James suffered from debilitating ulcerative colitis, which made his daily existence difficult and uncomfortable. Frustrated with traditional therapy, he set out on a journey to regain his health through nutritional modifications.

James selected a diet tailored to his condition after conducting extensive study and consulting with medical authorities. He concentrated on anti-inflammatory diets and avoided triggers that aggravated his symptoms. He gradually but steadily witnessed a transformative improvement.

The anguish of flare-ups subsided, replaced by a renewed vitality. James' patience and dedication to a specific diet not only helped him overcome ulcerative colitis, but also gave him the ability to take charge of his health. His tale inspired others facing similar issues, demonstrating the enormous influence that deliberate dietary decisions can have on chronic illness management.

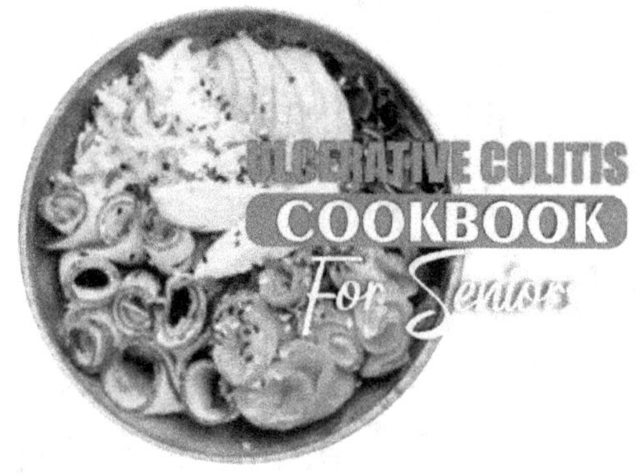

Chapter 1

The foods to eat or avoid on a ulcerative colitis diet to achieve optimum health.

Creating an ulcerative colitis cookbook for seniors involves careful consideration of foods that promote digestive health while avoiding those that may exacerbate symptoms. Optimum health for seniors with ulcerative colitis relies on a balanced and nourishing diet tailored to their specific needs. Here's a brief guide on foods to include and avoid in such a cookbook:

Foods to Include:

Low-Fiber Choices: Seniors with ulcerative colitis often benefit from low-fiber foods to minimize irritation. Incorporate well-cooked vegetables like carrots and zucchini, and choose refined grains such as white rice and white bread.

Lean Proteins: Opt for lean protein sources like poultry, fish, and eggs. These are easier to digest and provide essential amino acids crucial for overall health.

Probiotic-Rich Foods: Probiotics promote gut health and can be beneficial for those with ulcerative colitis. Include yogurt with live cultures, kefir, and fermented foods like sauerkraut to introduce beneficial bacteria.

Soft Fruits: Choose ripe, soft fruits like bananas, melons, and canned fruits without added sugars. These options are gentler on the digestive system.

Nutrient-Dense Soups: Prepare nutrient-rich soups using well-cooked vegetables, lean meats, and easily digestible grains like white rice. Soups can provide essential nutrients without putting excessive strain on the digestive tract.

Nut and Seed Butters: Smooth nut and seed butters are good sources of healthy fats and protein. They offer an alternative for seniors who may struggle with whole nuts and seeds.

Foods to Avoid:

High-Fiber Foods: Limit high-fiber foods such as raw vegetables, whole grains, and nuts as they can be challenging for seniors with ulcerative colitis to digest.

Dairy Products (if lactose intolerant): Seniors who are lactose intolerant may need to avoid dairy products or opt for lactose-free alternatives to prevent digestive discomfort.

Spicy and Greasy Foods: Spices and greasy foods can trigger inflammation and discomfort. It's advisable to minimize or avoid foods with high levels of spice and fat.

Certain Fruits and Vegetables: Some fruits and vegetables can be too rough on the digestive system. Avoid citrus fruits, berries with seeds, and cruciferous vegetables like broccoli and cauliflower.

Processed and Fried Foods: Processed foods often contain additives and preservatives that may aggravate symptoms. Additionally, fried foods can be harder to digest and may contribute to inflammation.

Caffeine and Alcohol: Both caffeine and alcohol can irritate the digestive tract. Encourage seniors to limit or avoid these substances to promote better gut health.

Creating a balanced ulcerative colitis cookbook for seniors involves tailoring meals to individual preferences and tolerances. It's crucial to consult with a healthcare professional or a registered dietitian to ensure that the proposed diet aligns with the specific needs of each senior with ulcerative colitis.

The core benefits of following a ulcerative colitis diet for seniors

1. Reduced Inflammation: A well-managed ulcerative colitis diet can help elders reduce inflammation in their digestive tracts, relieving symptoms and increasing overall comfort.

2. Nutrient Absorption: Tailoring the diet to the individual's needs allows improved absorption of vital nutrients, which is critical for sustaining

general health, particularly in seniors who may have higher nutrient requirements.

3. Weight Management: Customizing the diet can help seniors maintain a healthy weight while avoiding needless weight loss or gain caused by flare-ups or drug side effects.

4. Energy Levels: Eating a healthy diet will help stabilize energy levels, minimizing weariness and assisting seniors in keeping an active lifestyle.

5. Gastrointestinal Comfort: A correctly chosen diet can improve gastrointestinal comfort by minimizing the frequency and intensity of symptoms like abdominal pain and diarrhea.

6. Medication Support: Complementing medication with a specific diet may boost treatment effectiveness, perhaps eliminating the need for higher doses or additional medications.

7. Improved Quality of Life: By treating symptoms and supporting general well-being, a personalized ulcerative colitis diet can help seniors engage in daily activities more easily.

8. Complication Prevention: A healthy diet can help prevent ulcerative colitis complications such as malnutrition, anemia, and dehydration, so protecting seniors from further health risks.

Remember, it's essential for seniors to work closely with healthcare professionals and registered dietitians to create an individualized ulcerative colitis diet plan tailored to their specific needs and health conditions.

15

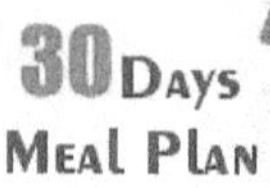

2024
LEONA BUTLER
ULCERATIVE COLITIS
COOKBOOK
For Seniors
Delicious And Healthy Dairy Free, Low Fiber Recipes To Relieve The Symptoms And Complications In Colitis Patients
14 BONUS
Weeks Meal
Planner Included
2000 DAYS RECIPES
30 Days
Meal Plan

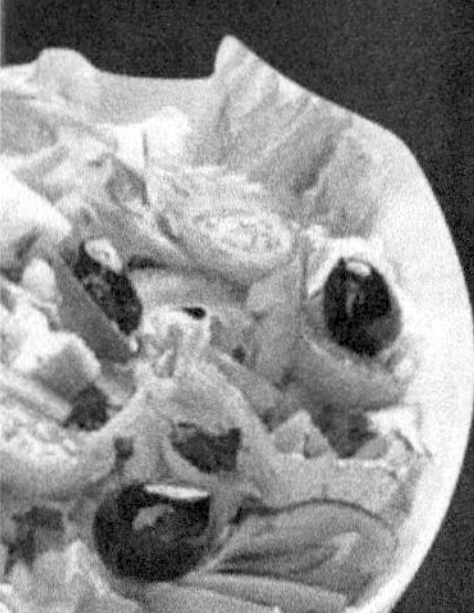

Chapter 2

How to follow a ulcerative colitis diet.

Low-Residue Diet: To avoid irritation, focus on readily digesting foods. Choose well-cooked veggies, peeled fruits, and refined grains.

Low-Fiber Options: Avoid high-fiber foods including nuts, seeds, and whole grains, as these might exacerbate symptoms.

Lean Proteins: Choose lean meats, poultry, fish, and eggs for a protein supply that is low in fat.

Dairy Alternatives: Somepeople with UC ma be lactose intolerant.
Consider lactose-free dairy and alternatives such as almond or soy milk.

17

Hydration: Stay hydrated to avoid dehydration from diarrhea. Water, herbal teas, and clear broths are excellent options.

Avoid Trigger Foods: Recognize and avoid foods that cause flare-ups. Spicy foods, coffee, alcohol, and certain artificial sweeteners are all common triggers.

Small, Frequent Meals: Eating smaller, more frequent meals can be better for the digestive system than larger meals.

Probiotics: To encourage a healthy balance of gut bacteria, consider eating probiotic-rich foods such as yogurt or taking supplements.

Limit Processed Foods: Avoid processed and fried foods, as they can be difficult to digest and may exacerbate symptoms.

Consult a Dietitian: Collaborate with a healthcare practitioner or a qualified dietitian to develop a personalized nutrition plan based on your unique needs and preferences.

Remember that individual reactions to meals might vary, so pay attention to your body's signals and speak with your healthcare provider for individualized advice.

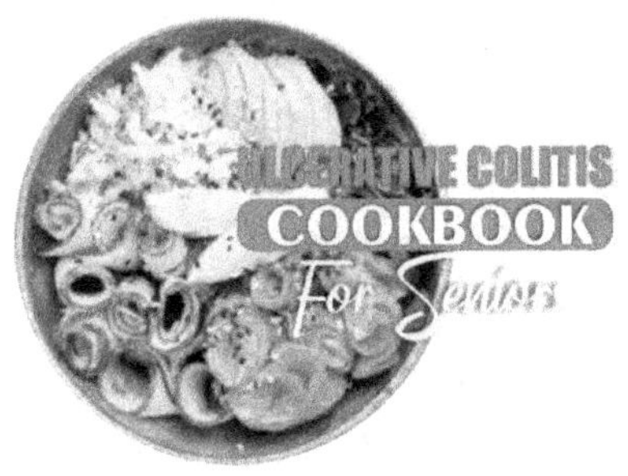

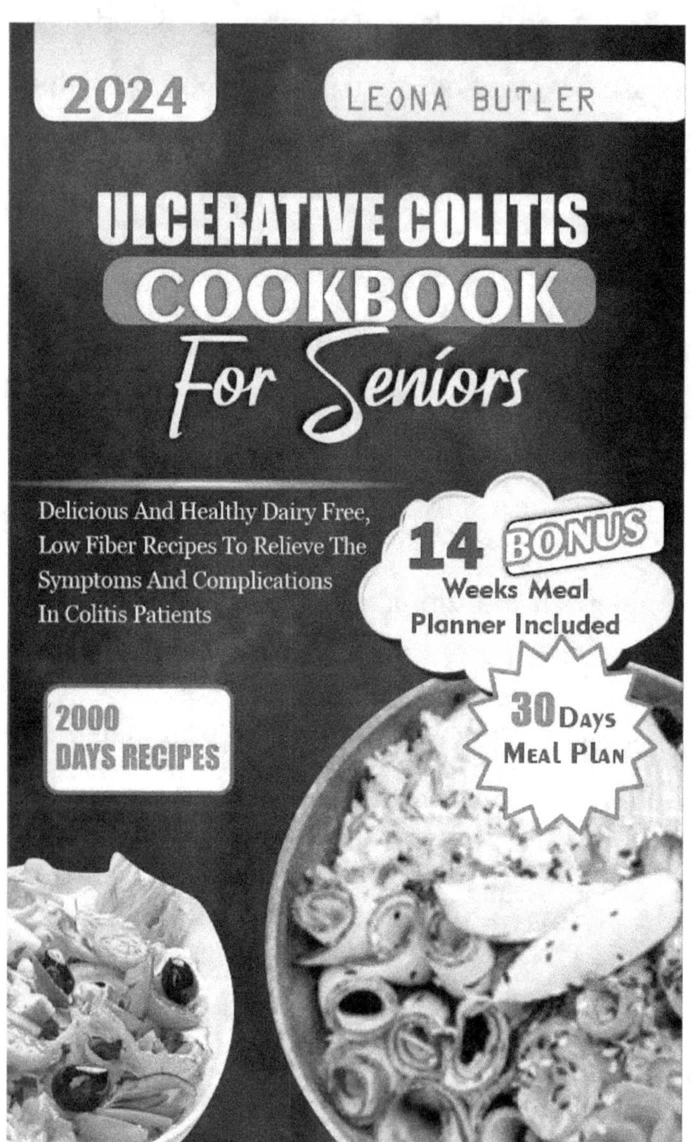

2024
LEONA BUTLER
ULCERATIVE COLITIS
COOKBOOK
For Seniors
Delicious And Healthy Dairy Free, Low Fiber Recipes To Relieve The Symptoms And Complications In Colitis Patients
14 BONUS
Weeks Meal Planner Included
2000 DAYS RECIPES
30 Days Meal Plan

Chapter 3

The complications of ulcerative colitis, if the right diet isn't adopted.

Ulcerative colitis can cause malnutrition, weight loss, and electrolyte abnormalities if not treated with a proper diet. Inflammation can worsen, resulting in severe stomach pain, diarrhea, and exhaustion. Long-term consequences could include intestinal perforation, strictures, and an increased risk of colon cancer.

Adopting a healthy diet that is low in specific fibers and irritants can help control symptoms and lower the chance of problems. Consultation with a healthcare practitioner or certified dietician is essential for tailored advice.

2024
LEONA BUTLER
ULCERATIVE COLITIS
COOKBOOK
For Seniors
Delicious And Healthy Dairy Free, Low Fiber Recipes To Relieve The Symptoms And Complications In Colitis Patients
14 BONUS
Weeks Meal
Planner Included
2000 DAYS RECIPES
30 Days Meal Plan

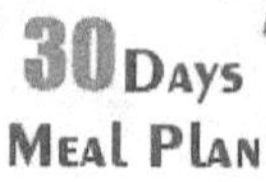

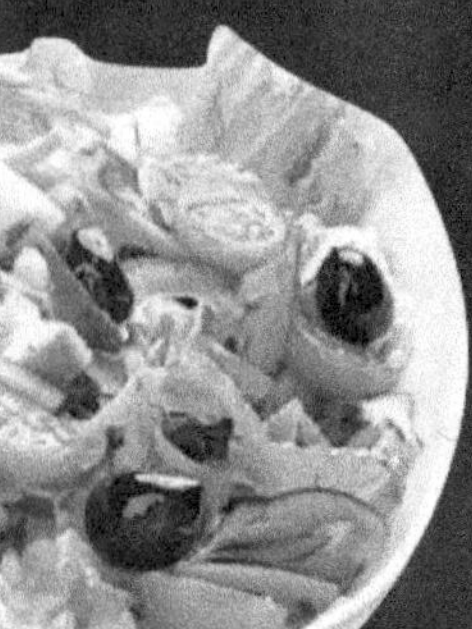

Chapter 4

Breakfast Recipes

1. Oatmeal with mashed banana and a sprinkle of ground flaxseeds.

Ingredients:

- 1/2 cup rolled oats

- 1 cup water or milk

- 1 ripe banana, mashed 1 tablespoon ground flaxseeds

Preparation:

1. In a saucepan, blend rolled oats with water (or milk).

2. Cook over medium heat, stirring occasionally, until the oats are tender (about 5 minutes).

3. Remove from heat and stir in the mashed banana.

4. Sprinkle ground flaxseeds on top and mix well.

5. Let it sit for a minute to thicken.

Enjoy your nutritious oatmeal!

Nutritional Value:

- Oats provide fiber and essential nutrients.

- Banana adds natural sweetness, potassium, and vitamins.

- Flaxseeds contribute omega-3 fatty acids and fiber.

Cooking Time: Approximately 5 minutes.

2. Scrambled eggs with spinach and a side of plain yogurt.

Ingredients:

- 2 eggs

- 1 cup fresh spinach, chopped

- Salt and pepper to taste 1/2 cup plain yogurt

Preparation:

1. In a bowl, whisk together the eggs and season with salt and pepper.

2. In a skillet, sauté chopped spinach until wilted.

3. Pour whisked eggs over the spinach and scramble until cooked to your liking.

4. Serve with a side of plain yogurt.

Nutritional Value:

- Eggs provide protein and essential amino acids.

- Spinach offers vitamins, minerals, and antioxidants.

- Yogurt adds probiotics and calcium.

Cooking Time: Approximately 7-10 minutes.

Enjoy your wholesome meals!

3. Brown Rice Porridge with Cooked Apples and Honey

Ingredients:

- cup brown rice

- cups water
- cup milk (dairy or plant-based)
- apples, peeled and diced
- 2 tablespoons honey

Preparation:

1. Rinse the brown rice thoroughly.
2. In a pot, combine rinsed rice, water, and milk. Bring to a boil.
3. Reduce heat to low, cover, and simmer for 45-50 minutes or until rice is tender.
4. In a separate pan, cook diced apples until soft.
5. Once the porridge is ready, spoon it into bowls, top with cooked apples, and drizzle honey.

Serve warm.

Nutritional Value:

- Brown rice is a good source of fiber, minerals, and vitamins.
- Apples provide dietary fiber and various antioxidants.

- Honey adds natural sweetness and may have antibacterial properties.

Cooking Time: Approximately 50 minutes.

4. Quinoa and Vegetable Stir-Fry with Soft-Cooked Eggs

Ingredients:

- cup quinoa
- cups water or vegetable broth
- 2 cups mixed veggies (such as bell peppers, broccoli, and carrots)
- 2 tablespoons soy sauce
- 2 tablespoons oil
- 4 eggs

Preparation:

1. Rinse quinoa under cold water.
2. In a saucepan, combine the quinoa and water (or broth). Bring to a boil, then simmer for 15-20

minutes until quinoa is cooked and liquid is absorbed.

3. In a wok or pan, heat oil and stir-fry mixed vegetables until tender. Add cooked quinoa to the vegetables, pour soy sauce, and toss until well combined.

4. In a separate pan, cook eggs to your liking (soft-cooked is recommended). Serve the quinoa and vegetable stir-fry in bowls, topped with soft-cooked eggs.

Nutritional Value:

- Quinoa is rich in protein, fiber, and various nutrients.

- Mixed vegetables offer vitamins and minerals.

- Eggs supply additional protein and critical amino acids.

Cooking Time:

Approximately 25-30 minutes.

Ingredients:

- 1 cup Greek yogurt

- 1/2 cup granola

- 1 cup mixed berries (strawberries, blueberries, raspberries)

- kiwi, peeled and sliced

- tablespoons honey

- 1/4 cup chopped nuts (almonds, walnuts, or your choice)

Preparation:

1. In a serving glass or bowl, start with a layer of Greek yogurt at the bottom. Top the yogurt with a layer of granola.

2. Place a generous layer of mixed berries on the granola.

3. Add a layer of sliced kiwi over the berries.

4. Drizzle honey evenly over the fruit layer.

5. Continue layering until you reach the top of the glass or bowl.

6. Finish with a sprinkle of chopped nuts for added crunch.

Nutritional Value (per serving):

- Calories: Approximately 350-400 kcal

- Protein: 20g

- Carbohydrates: 45g

- Fat: 15g

- Fiber: 8g

Cooking Time:

No cooking required, as it's a no-cook recipe. The time needed for preparation is around 10 minutes.

Enjoy your healthy Greek yogurt parfait!

Ingredients:

- 1 ripe banana

- 1 cup almond milk

- 1 tablespoon nut butter (e.g., almond or peanut butter)

Preparation:

1. Peel and slice the ripe banana.

2. In a blender, combine the sliced banana, almond milk, and nut butter. Blend at high speed until smooth and thoroughly incorporated.

Quantity/Measurement:

- 1 ripe banana

- 1 cup almond milk

- 1 tablespoon nut butter

Nutritional Value (approximate):

- Calories: Around 250

- Protein: 6g

- Fat: 15g

- Carbohydrates: 30g

- Fiber: 5g

- Sugar: 15g

Cooking Time:

5 minutes

Enjoy your nutritious and delicious smoothie!

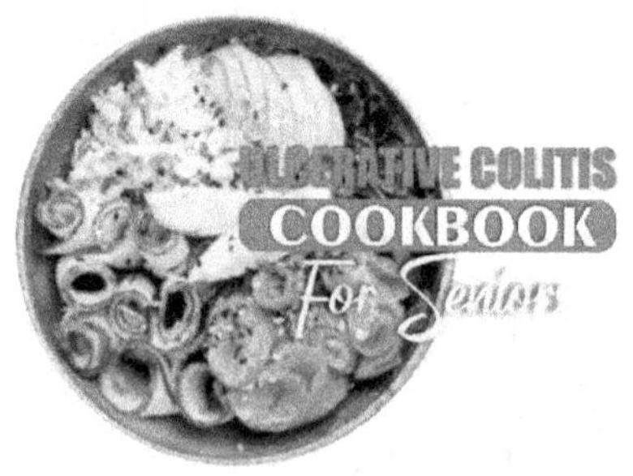

Ingredients:

- 4 medium-sized sweet potatoes

- 1 cup plain yogurt

- Fresh chives, chopped Salt and pepper to taste

Preparation:

1. Preheat the oven to 400°F (200°C).

2. Wash and scrub the sweet potatoes thoroughly.

3. Pierce each sweet potato with a fork a few times to allow steam to escape during baking.

4. Place the sweet potatoes on a baking sheet and bake for 45-60 minutes or until tender.

5. In the meantime, mix the plain yogurt with a pinch of salt in a bowl. Once the sweet

33

potatoes are done, slice each one open and fluff the insides with a fork.

6. Add a dollop of yogurt on top of each sweet potato.

7. Sprinkle chopped chives over the yogurt and season with salt and pepper to taste.

Nutritional Value (per serving):

- Calories: Approximately 200-250 kcal

- Protein: 5g

- Carbohydrates: 45g

- Dietary Fiber: 7g

- Sugars: 12g

- Fat: 2g

- Calcium: 150mg

- Iron: 2mg Vitamin C: 30mg

Cooking Time:

45-60 minutes (baking the sweet potatoes)

Ingredients:

- 1 cup cottage cheese
- 1 cup sliced peaches
- A handful of walnuts

Preparation:

1. In a bowl, combine 1 cup of cottage cheese.
2. Add 1 cup of sliced peaches to the cottage cheese.
3. Toss in a handful of walnuts.
4. Gently mix the ingredients until well combined.

Nutritional Value (approximate):

- Calories: 400
- Protein: 25g
- Fat: 20g

- Carbohydrates: 30g

- Fiber: 5g

Cooking Time: 5 minutes

9. Buckwheat pancakes with pureed berries as a topping.

Ingredients:

- 1 cup buckwheat flour

- cup all-purpose flour

- tablespoons sugar

- tablespoon baking powder

- 1/2 teaspoon salt

- large eggs

- 1 3/4 cups milk

- 1/4 cup melted butter

- 1 cup mixed berries (for puree and topping)

Preparation:

1. In a large mixing bowl, whisk together the buckwheat flour, all-purpose flour, sugar, baking powder, and salt.
2. In a separate bowl, beat the eggs and then add the milk and melted butter. Mix well.
3. Pour the wet ingredients into the dry ingredients and mix just until mixed. Allow the batter to rest for 5–10 minutes.
4. While the batter rests, puree the mixed berries in a blender until smooth. Heat a griddle or skillet over medium heat. Grease with a small amount of butter or oil.
5. Pour 1/4 cup of batter onto the griddle for each pancake. Cook until bubbles appear on the surface, then flip and finish till golden brown.
6. Repeat until all the batter is used.

Nutritional Value (per serving):

- Calories: Approximately 220 kcal

- Protein: 6g

- Fat: 8g

- Carbohydrates: 32g

- Fiber: 3g

- Sugars: 8g

Cooking Time:

Total: Approximately 20 minutes

Enjoy your nutritious buckwheat pancakes with pureed berry topping!

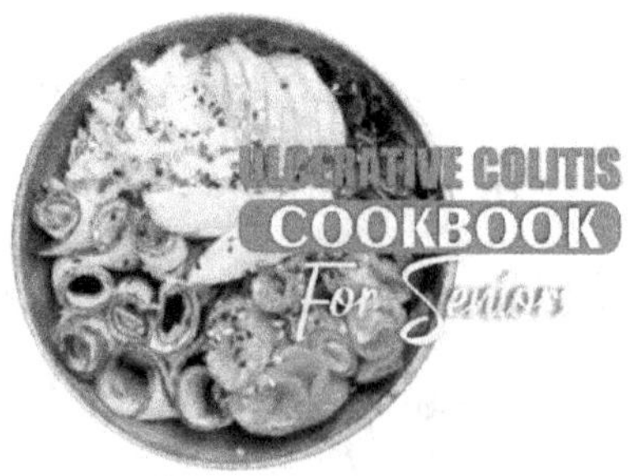

Ingredients:

- 2 large eggs

- 2 cups fresh spinach

- 1 slice whole-grain bread Salt and pepper to taste

Preparation:

1. Heat a small pot of water to a slow boil.

2. Carefully add the eggs to the boiling water and simmer for 4-5 minutes for soft-boiled eggs.

3. While the eggs are cooking, steam the spinach for 2-3 minutes until wilted.

4. Toast the whole-grain bread slice to your preference.

5. Once the eggs are done, transfer them to a bowl of cold water for easy peeling.

6. Place the steamed spinach on a plate, add the peeled soft-boiled eggs, and serve with the whole-grain toast.

7. Season with salt and pepper to taste.

Nutritional Value (approximate):

- Calories: 320

- Protein: 18g

- Fat: 14g

- Carbohydrates: 30g

- Fiber: 7g

Cooking Time: 10-15 minutes

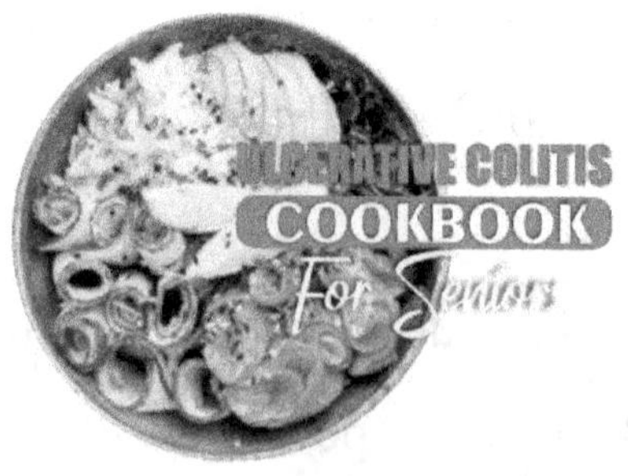

Lunch recipes

1. Grilled chicken with steamed carrots and mashed sweet potatoes.

Grilled Chicken:

Ingredients:

- 2 boneless, skinless chicken breasts
- 1 tablespoon olive oil
- 1 teaspoon salt
- 1 teaspoon black pepper
- 1 teaspoon garlic powder
- 1 teaspoon paprika

Preparation:

1. Preheat grill to medium-high heat. Rub chicken breasts with olive oil.

2. Season with salt and pepper, garlic powder, and paprika.

3. Grill for 6–8 minutes per side, or until the internal temperature reaches 165°F.

Nutritional Value (per serving):

- Calories: 250

- Protein: 30g

- Fat: 12g

- Carbohydrates: 2g

- Fiber: 1g

Steamed Carrots:

Ingredients:

- 1 cup baby carrots

- Water for steaming 1/2 teaspoon salt

Preparation:

- Place carrots in a steamer basket.
- Steam for 8-10 minutes until tender.
- Sprinkle with salt before serving.

Nutritional Value (per serving):

- Calories: 35
- Protein: 1g
- Fat: 0g
- Carbohydrates: 8g
- Fiber: 2g

Mashed Sweet Potatoes:

Ingredients:

- 2 large sweet potatoes, peeled and diced
- 2 tablespoons butter
- 1/4 cup milk
- Salt and pepper to taste Preparation:

- Boil sweet potatoes until fork-tender, about 15-20 minutes.
- Drain and mash with butter and milk.
- Season with salt and pepper.

Nutritional Value (per serving):

- Calories: 200
- Protein: 2g
- Fat: 8g
- Carbohydrates: 30g
- Fiber: 4g

Cooking Time:

Grilled Chicken: 15-20 minutes

Steamed Carrots: 8-10 minutes

Mashed Sweet Potatoes: 20-25 minutes (including boiling time)

Ingredients:

- Salmon Fillets (4 pieces): Approximately 6 oz each.

- Quinoa (1 cup): Rinsed thoroughly.

- Zucchini (2 medium-sized): Sliced.

- Olive Oil (2 tablespoons): Divided.

- Lemon (1): Sliced for garnish.

- Garlic (2 cloves): Minced.

- Dill (1 tablespoon): Fresh, chopped.

- Salt and Pepper: To taste.

For the Quinoa:

- Rinse quinoa under cold water.

- Combine quinoa with 2 cups of water in a saucepan, bring to a boil, then simmer for 15-20 minutes until water is absorbed.

For the Roasted Zucchini:

- Preheat oven to 400°F (200°C).

- Toss zucchini slices with 1 tablespoon olive oil, salt, and pepper.

- Spread on a baking sheet and roast for 20-25 minutes, turning halfway through.

For the Baked Salmon:

- Preheat oven to 375°F (190°C).

- Season salmon with salt, pepper, minced garlic, and dill.

- Place salmon on a baking sheet lined with parchment paper.

- Drizzle with remaining olive oil and lay lemon slices on top.

- Bake for 15-20 minutes or until salmon flakes easily with a fork.

Nutritional Value (per serving):

- Calories: Approximately 500-600 kcal

- Protein: Around 35-40g

- Healthy Fats: 20-25g

- Carbohydrates: 35-40g

Cooking Time:

Total: Approximately 45-50 minutes.

3. Turkey and vegetable stir-fry with brown rice.

Ingredients:

- lb (450g) turkey breast, thinly sliced

- cups (400g) mixed vegetables (broccoli, bell peppers, snap peas, carrots), chopped

- cup (185g) brown rice

- tablespoons (30ml) soy sauce

- 1 tablespoon (15ml) sesame oil

- tablespoon (15ml) olive oil

- cloves garlic, minced

- 1 teaspoon (5g) ginger, grated

- Salt and pepper to taste

- Green onions for garnish (optional) Sesame seeds for garnish (optional)

Nutritional Value:

- Approximate per serving:

- Calories: 450

- Protein: 30g

- Carbohydrates: 45g

- Fat: 15g

- Fiber: 5g

Preparation:

1. Cook brown rice according to package instructions.

2. Warm olive oil in a large skillet or wok over medium-high heat.

3. Add sliced turkey and cook until browned, approximately 4-5 minutes.

4. Remove turkey from the skillet and set aside.

5. In the same skillet, add sesame oil, garlic, and ginger. Sauté for 1-2 minutes.

6. Add mixed vegetables to the skillet and stir-fry until crisp-tender, about 5-7 minutes.

7. Return cooked turkey to the skillet, pour in soy sauce, and toss until well combined. Season with salt and pepper to taste.

8. Serve the stir-fry over cooked brown rice.

9. If desired, garnish with green onion and sesame seeds.

Cooking Time:

Total: Approximately 30 minutes.

4. Spinach and feta omelette with a side of roasted bell peppers.

Ingredients:

- 3 large eggs
- 1 cup fresh spinach, chopped
- 1/4 cup feta cheese, crumbled
- 1/2 cup bell peppers, sliced
- Salt and pepper to taste
- 1 tablespoon olive oil

Nutritional Value (approximate per serving):

- Calories: 350
- Protein: 20g
- Fat: 25g
- Carbohydrates: 10g
- Fiber: 3g

Preparation:

1. In a mixing dish, whisk together the eggs. Add a pinch of salt and pepper.
2. Heat olive oil in a non-stick skillet over medium heat.
3. Add the chopped spinach to the skillet and sauté for 1-2 minutes until wilted.
4. Pour the whisked eggs over the spinach, ensuring an even spread.
5. Sprinkle crumbled feta evenly over the eggs.
6. Allow the omelette to cook for 3-4 minutes until the edges set.
7. Carefully flip the omelette over and cook for another 2-3 minutes on the other side.
8. In a separate pan, roast the bell peppers with a dash of olive oil until slightly charred.
9. Serve the spinach and feta omelette hot, with a side of roasted bell peppers.

Cooking Time:

Omelette: 7-8 minutes

Roasted Bell Peppers: 5-6 minutes

Enjoy your nutritious and delicious meal!

5. Lentil soup with whole-grain toast.

Ingredients:

- 1 cup dried lentils
- 4 cups vegetable broth
- onion, finely chopped
- carrots, diced
- celery stalks, chopped
- cloves garlic, minced
- 1 can (14 oz) diced tomatoes
- 1 teaspoon cumin
- 1 teaspoon paprika
- Salt and pepper to taste 4 slices whole-grain bread

Nutritional Value:

- Lentils: Rich in protein, fiber, and various nutrients.
- Vegetables: Provide essential vitamins and minerals.
- Whole-grain bread: High in fiber, vitamins, and minerals.

Preparation:

1. Rinse lentils under cold water and drain.
2. In a large pot, cook the onions, carrots, and celery until tender.
3. Add garlic, cumin, and paprika; cook for an additional minute.
4. Pour in vegetable broth, lentils, and diced tomatoes. Bring to a boil.
5. Reduce heat, cover, and simmer for 25-30 minutes or until lentils are tender.
6. Season with salt and pepper to taste.

7. While the soup simmers, toast whole-grain bread slices.

8. Serve lentil soup hot, accompanied by whole-grain toast. Cooking Time: 25-30 minutes for the soup.

Enjoy your wholesome lentil soup with nutritious whole-grain toast!

6. Grilled shrimp salad with mixed greens and a light vinaigrette.

Ingredients:

- 1 pound (450g) of large shrimp, peeled and deveined
- 6 cups mixed greens (spinach, arugula, and romaine)
- 1 cup cherry tomatoes, halved
- cucumber, sliced

- 1/4 cup red onion, thinly sliced 1/4 cup feta cheese, crumbled For the Vinaigrette:

- 1/4 cup olive oil

- tablespoons balsamic vinegar

- 1 teaspoon Dijon mustard

- 1 clove garlic, minced Salt and pepper to taste

Preparation:

1. Preheat grill to medium-high heat.

2. In a bowl, toss shrimp with olive oil, salt, and pepper.

3. Grill shrimp for 2-3 minutes per side until opaque and cooked through.

4. In a large salad bowl, combine mixed greens, cherry tomatoes, cucumber, red onion, and grilled shrimp.

5. In a small bowl, whisk together olive oil, balsamic vinegar, Dijon mustard, garlic, salt, and pepper to create the vinaigrette.

6. Pour the vinaigrette over the salad and gently toss to coat evenly.

7. Sprinkle crumbled feta cheese over the top.

8. Serve immediately and enjoy your delicious grilled shrimp salad!

Nutritional Value (approximate per serving):

- Calories: 350

- Protein: 25g

- Carbohydrates: 12g

- Fat: 24g

- Fiber: 4g

Cooking Time:

Grilling shrimp: 6-8 minutes

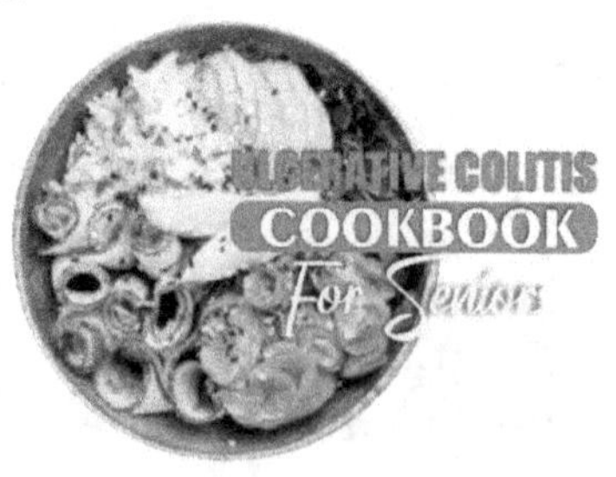

7. Baked cod with sautéed spinach and quinoa.

Ingredients:

- 4 cod fillets (about 6 oz each)

- 2 cups quinoa

- 4 cups fresh spinach

- 2 tablespoons olive oil

- 2 cloves garlic, minced

- 1 lemon, sliced Salt and pepper to taste

Preparation:

1. Preheat the oven to 375°F (190°C).

2. Rinse the quinoa under cold water.In a saucepan, combine quinoa and 4 cups water. Bring to a boil, then decrease heat, cover, and cook for 15-20 minutes, or until the water is absorbed.

3. Place cod fillets on a baking sheet lined with parchment paper. Season with salt and pepper.

4. Lay lemon slices on top of the fillets.

5. Bake cod in the preheated oven for 15-20 minutes or until it flakes easily with a fork. In a large skillet, heat the olive oil over medium heat. Add the minced garlic and cook until fragrant.

6. Add fresh spinach to the skillet and sauté until wilted, about 3-5 minutes.

7. Serve baked cod over a bed of cooked quinoa and sautéed spinach. Drizzle with lemon juice from the baked slices.

Enjoy your nutritious meal!

Nutritional Value (approximate per serving):

- Calories: 500
- Protein: 40g
- Carbohydrates: 45g
- Fat: 18g
- Fiber: 6g

Cooking Time: 35-40 minutes

8. Turkey and vegetable wrap with a gluten-free tortilla.

8. Turkey and vegetable wrap with a gluten-free tortilla.

Ingredients:

- 1 gluten-free tortilla

- 4 oz (about 115g) turkey breast, thinly sliced

- 1/2 cup (about 75g) cherry tomatoes, halved

- 1/2 cup (about 75g) cucumber, thinly sliced

- 1/4 cup (about 30g) red bell pepper, thinly sliced

- 2 tbsp (about 30g) hummus

- 1 cup (about 40g) mixed salad greens Salt and pepper to taste

Preparation:

1. Lay the gluten-free tortilla flat on a clean surface.

2. Spread the hummus evenly over the entire surface of the tortilla.

3. Place the thinly sliced turkey breast in the center of the tortilla, leaving space around the edges.

Sprinkle the cherry tomatoes, cucumber, red bell pepper, and mixed salad greens over the turkey.

4. Season with salt and pepper to taste.

5. Fold the sides of the tortilla inwards and then roll it up tightly from the bottom to form a wrap. Slice the wrap in half diagonally for easier handling.

Nutritional Value:

- Calories: Approximately 400 kcal

- Protein: 25g

- Carbohydrates: 40g

- Dietary Fiber: 6g

- Sugars: 4g

- Fat: 16g

- Saturated Fat: 3g

- Cholesterol: 40mg

- Sodium: 700mg

Ingredients:

- medium-sized butternut squash

- boneless, skinless chicken breasts

- 2 tablespoons olive oil

- Salt and pepper to taste

- 1 teaspoon garlic powder

- 1 teaspoon dried thyme 1/2 cup chicken broth

Preparation:

1. Preheat the oven to 400°F (200°C).

2. Peel, seed, and chop the butternut squash into 1-inch pieces.

3. Place the butternut squash cubes on a baking sheet, drizzle with 1 tablespoon of olive oil, and sprinkle with salt and pepper. Cook in the oven for 25-30 minutes, or until tender.

4. While the squash is roasting, season the chicken breasts with salt, pepper, garlic powder, and dried thyme.

5. In a skillet, heat the remaining 1 tablespoon of olive oil over medium-high heat. Add the seasoned chicken breasts and sear for 3-4 minutes on each side until golden brown. Reduce heat to medium, pour in the chicken broth, cover the skillet, and simmer for about 15 minutes or until the chicken is cooked through.

6. Once the butternut squash is roasted, transfer it to a bowl and mash it with a fork or potato masher.

7. Slice the cooked chicken breasts.

8. Serve the mashed butternut squash topped with sliced roasted chicken breasts.

Nutritional Value:

- Butternut Squash: Rich in vitamins A and C, fiber, and potassium.
- Chicken Breast: High in protein, low in fat.

Cooking Time:

Roasting Butternut Squash: 25-30 minutes

Cooking Chicken Breasts: 15 minutes

10. Quinoa and roasted vegetable bowl with a touch of olive oil.

Ingredients:

- cup quinoa
- cups mixed vegetables (e.g., bell peppers, zucchini, cherry tomatoes)
- 2 tablespoons olive oil Salt and pepper to taste

Preparation:

1. Rinse 1 cup of quinoa thoroughly under cold water.

2. In a saucepan, combine the quinoa with 2 cups of water. Bring to a boil, then decrease heat, cover, and cook for 15-20 minutes, or until the water is absorbed.

3. Preheat the oven to 400°F (200°C).

4. Chop the mixed vegetables into bite-sized pieces.

5. Toss the vegetables with 1 tablespoon of olive oil, salt, and pepper on a baking sheet.

6. Roast the vegetables in a warm oven for 20-25 minutes, or until soft and faintly caramelized.

7. While the vegetables are roasting, fluff the cooked quinoa with a fork.

8. Once the vegetables are done, assemble the bowl by placing a portion of quinoa in the center and arranging the roasted vegetables around it.

9. Drizzle the last tablespoon of olive oil over the bowl. Season with more salt and pepper to taste.

Nutritional Value (per serving):

- Calories: Approximately 400-450 kcal

- Protein: 10g

- Fat: 18g

- Carbohydrates: 55g

- Fiber: 8g

Cooking Time: Approximately 45-50 minutes (including prep and roasting time)

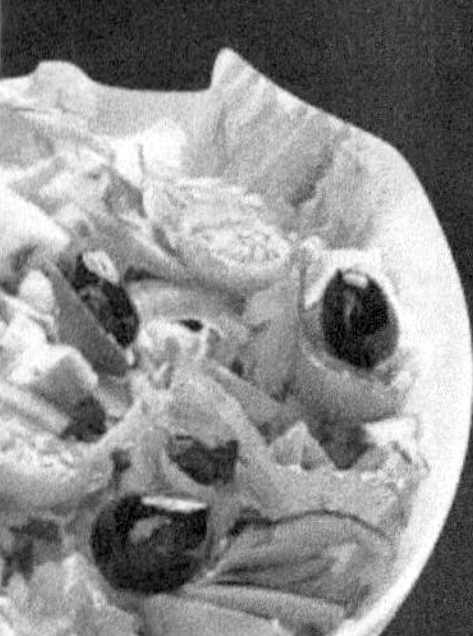

2024
LEONA BUTLER
ULCERATIVE COLITIS
COOKBOOK
For Seniors
Delicious And Healthy Dairy Free,
Low Fiber Recipes To Relieve The
Symptoms And Complications
In Colitis Patients
14 BONUS
Weeks Meal
Planner Included
2000
DAYS RECIPES
30 Days
Meal Plan

Dinner Recipes

1.Baked Salmon with Quinoa and Steamed Vegetables

Ingredients:

- 4 salmon fillets (6 oz each)

- cup quinoa

- cups mixed vegetables (broccoli, carrots, and snap peas)

- 2 tablespoons olive oil

- 2 cloves garlic, minced

- 1 lemon, sliced

- Salt and pepper to taste

- Fresh herbs (parsley or dill) for garnish

Nutritional Value (per serving):

- Calories: Approximately 500

- Protein: 30g

- Fat: 22g

- Carbohydrates: 45g

- Fiber: 7g

Preparation:

1. Preheat the oven to 400°F (200°C).

2. Rinse quinoa under cold water. In a saucepan, combine 2 cups of water, quinoa, and a pinch of salt. Bring to a boil, then reduce heat, cover, and let simmer for 15 minutes.

3. Season the salmon fillets with salt and pepper. Arrange them on a baking sheet lined with parchment paper.

4. In a small bowl, mix olive oil and minced garlic. Brush the salmon fillets with this mixture and place lemon slices on top.

5. Bake salmon in the preheated oven for 12-15 minutes or until cooked through and flaky.

While the salmon is baking, steam mixed vegetables for about 5-7 minutes until tender but still crisp.

6. Fluff the cooked quinoa with a fork and serve as a base on each plate.

7. Place a salmon fillet on the quinoa and arrange steamed vegetables on the side. Garnish with fresh herbs and more lemon slices, if preferred.

Cooking Time:

Salmon: 12-15 minutes

Quinoa: 15 minutes

Steamed Vegetables: 5-7 minutes

2. Mashed Sweet Potatoes with Grilled Chicken and Green Beans:

Ingredients:

- 4 medium-sized sweet potatoes
- 4 boneless, skinless chicken breasts
- 1 pound green beans, trimmed
- 1/4 cup olive oil Salt and pepper to taste

Preparation:

1. Peel and chop the sweet potatoes into cubes.
2. Boil the sweet potatoes until fork-tender, then mash them with a fork or potato masher. Season with salt and pepper.
3. Season chicken breasts with salt and pepper, then grill until cooked through, approximately 6-8 minutes per side.
4. In a separate pan, sauté green beans in olive oil until they are crisp-tender.

5. Serve the grilled chicken on a bed of mashed sweet potatoes, with a side of green beans.

Nutritional Value:

- Calories: Approximately 400 per serving

- Protein: 30g

- Carbohydrates: 40g

- Fat: 15g

- Fiber: 8g

Cooking Time:

Sweet Potatoes: 20 minutes

Grilled Chicken: 15 minutes Green Beans: 8-10 minutes

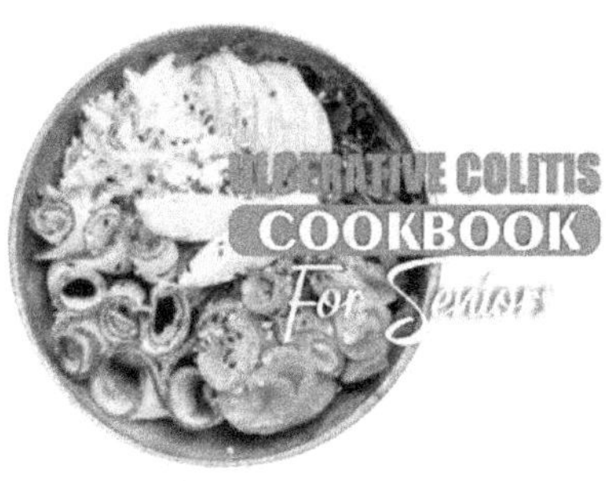

3. Turkey and Vegetable Stir-Fry with Brown Rice:

Ingredients:

- pound lean ground turkey
- cups mixed vegetables (bell peppers, broccoli, carrots)
- 1 cup brown rice
- 3 tablespoons soy sauce
- 2 tablespoons sesame oil
- 2 cloves garlic, minced 1 teaspoon ginger, grated

Preparation:

1. Cook brown rice according to package instructions.
2. In a large skillet, cook ground turkey until browned. Drain excess fat.
3. Add minced garlic and grated ginger to the skillet, sauté for 1-2 minutes.

4. Add mixed vegetables to the skillet, stir-fry until they are tender-crisp.

5. Pour soy sauce and sesame oil over the mixture, stir to combine.

6. Serve the stir-fry over cooked brown rice.

Nutritional Value:

- Calories: Approximately 450 per serving

- Protein: 25g

- Carbohydrates: 50g

- Fat: 18g

- Fiber: 6g Cooking Time:

- Brown Rice: 45 minutes

- Turkey Stir-Fry: 15 minutes

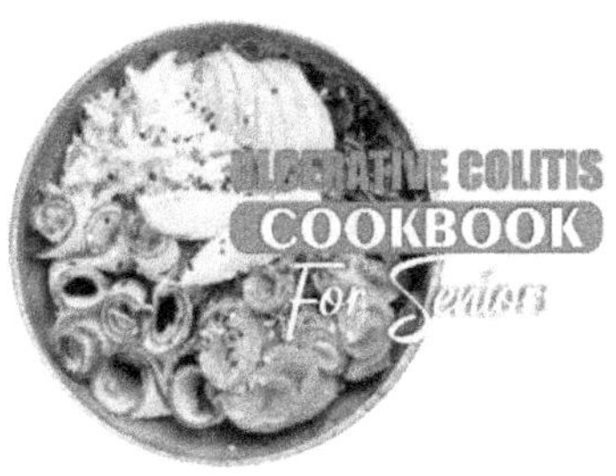

4. Grilled Tilapia with Lemon Herb Quinoa and Roasted Zucchini Grilled Tilapia with Lemon Herb

Quinoa and Roasted Zucchini:

Ingredients:

- 4 tilapia fillets (about 6 oz each)
- cup quinoa
- cups water
- lemon (juiced and zested)
- tablespoons olive oil
- 2 cloves garlic (minced)
- teaspoon dried thyme
- Salt and pepper to taste
- medium-sized zucchinis (sliced)
- Fresh parsley for garnish

Nutritional Value (per serving):

- Calories: ~400

- Protein: ~30g

- Carbohydrates: ~30g

- Fat: ~18g

- Fiber: ~4g

Preparation:

1. Preheat the grill and oven to medium-high heat.

2. Rinse quinoa under cold water. In a saucepan, mix the quinoa, water, and a touch of salt. Bring to a boil, then reduce heat and simmer for 15-20 minutes.

3. In a bowl, mix olive oil, lemon juice, lemon zest, minced garlic, dried thyme, salt, and pepper.

4. Coat tilapia fillets with this mixture.

5. Grill tilapia for 4-5 minutes per side until cooked through.

6. While grilling, toss zucchini slices with olive oil, salt, and pepper. Roast in the oven for 15-20 minutes.

7. Fluff quinoa with a fork and add chopped fresh parsley.

8. Serve grilled tilapia over lemon herb quinoa, with roasted zucchini on the side.

Cooking Time:

Grilling Tilapia: 8-10 minutes

Roasting Zucchini: 15-20 minutes

Cooking Quinoa: 15-20 minutes

Chicken and Rice Soup with Carrots and Spinach:

Ingredients:

- 1 lb chicken breasts (cooked and shredded)

- 1 cup white rice

- 8 cups chicken broth

- 2 carrots (peeled and diced)

- 2 cups fresh spinach leaves

- onion (chopped)

- cloves garlic (minced)

- teaspoon dried thyme

- Salt and pepper to taste

- tablespoons olive oil

Nutritional Value (per serving):

- Calories: ~300

- Protein: ~25g

- Carbohydrates: ~30g

- Fat: ~8g

- Fiber: ~3g

Preparation:

1. Cook chicken breasts and shred them.

2. In a large pot, sauté chopped onions and minced garlic in olive oil until softened.

3. Add chicken broth, diced carrots, rice, shredded chicken, dried thyme, salt, and pepper. Bring to a boil.

4. Reduce the heat to a simmer for 15-20 minutes, or until the rice is done.

5. Add fresh spinach leaves and simmer for an additional 5 minutes until wilted.

6. Adjust seasoning if needed.

Cooking Time:

Preparing Chicken: 15-20 minutes

Cooking Soup: 30-35 minutes Enjoy your nutritious meals!

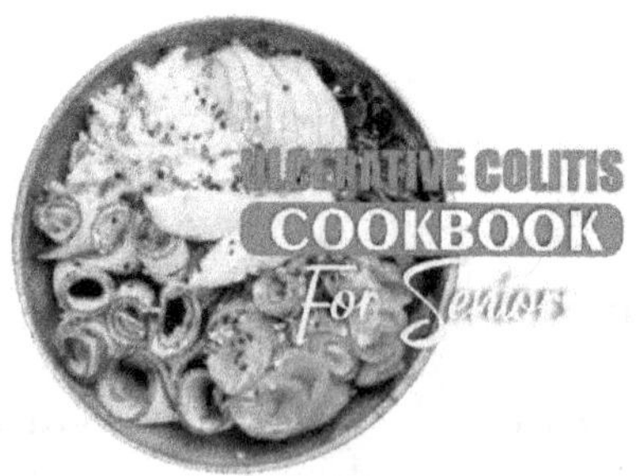

5. Chicken and Rice Soup with Carrots and Spinach

Ingredients:

- 1 lb chicken breasts (cooked and shredded)

- 1 cup white rice

- 8 cups chicken broth

- 2 carrots (peeled and diced)

- 2 cups fresh spinach leaves

- onion (chopped)

- cloves garlic (minced)

- teaspoon dried thyme

- Salt and pepper to taste

- tablespoons olive oil

Nutritional Value (per serving):

- Calories: ~300

- Protein: ~25g

- Carbohydrates: ~30g

- Fat: ~8g

- Fiber: ~3g

Preparation:

- Cook chicken breasts and shred them.

- In a large pot, sauté chopped onions and minced garlic in olive oil until softened.

- Add chicken broth, diced carrots, rice, shredded chicken, dried thyme, salt, and pepper. Bring to a boil.

- Reduce the heat to a simmer for 15-20 minutes, or until the rice is done.

- Add fresh spinach leaves and simmer for an additional 5 minutes until wilted.

- Adjust seasoning if needed.

Cooking Time:

Preparing Chicken: 15-20 minutes Cooking Soup: 30-35 minutes Enjoy your nutritious meals!

6. Baked Cod with Cilantro Lime Rice and Steamed Asparagus gus:

Ingredients:

For Baked Cod:

- 4 cod fillets (about 6 oz each)

- 2 tablespoons olive oil

- 1 teaspoon garlic powder

- 1 teaspoon paprika

- Salt and pepper to taste

- Fresh lemon wedges for serving

For Cilantro Lime Rice:

- cup long-grain white rice

- cups water

- 1/4 cup fresh cilantro, chopped

- Juice of 1 lime

- Salt to taste

For Steamed Asparagus:

- 1 bunch asparagus, trimmed

- 1 tablespoon olive oil Salt and pepper to taste

Preparation:

Baked Cod:

- Preheat the oven to 400°F (200°C).

- Place cod fillets on a baking sheet lined with parchment paper.

- Drizzle olive oil over the cod and sprinkle with garlic powder, paprika, salt, and pepper.

- Bake for 15-20 minutes, or until the fish flaked easily with a fork.

- Serve with fresh lemon wedges.

- To make Cilantro Lime Rice, rinse the rice under cold water until clear.

- In a saucepan, combine rice, water, and a pinch of salt. Bring to a boil.

- Reduce heat, cover, and simmer for 18-20 minutes or until rice is tender.
- Fluff the rice with a fork, then stir in chopped cilantro and lime juice.

Steamed Asparagus:

- Steam asparagus until crisp-tender, about 4-5 minutes.
- Heat olive oil in a pan, add steamed asparagus, and sauté for 2 minutes.
- Season with salt and pepper.

Nutritional Value (per serving):

- Baked Cod: Approx. 250 calories, 30g protein, 12g fat, 2g carbs
- Cilantro Lime Rice: Approx. 200 calories, 4g protein, 2g fat, 40g carbs Steamed Asparagus: Approx. 50 calories, 4g protein, 4g fat, 6g carbs

Cooking Time:

- Baked Cod: 15-20 minutes

- Cilantro Lime Rice: 20 minutes

- Steamed Asparagus: 4-5 minutes

7. Quinoa Salad with Grilled Shrimp, Cherry Tomatoes, and Avocado

Ingredients:

- 1 cup quinoa

- 1 pound large shrimp, peeled and deveined

- pint cherry tomatoes, halved

- avocados, diced

- 1/4 cup olive oil

- 2 tablespoons balsamic vinegar

- 1 teaspoon Dijon mustard

- Salt and pepper to taste Fresh parsley for garnish

For the Quinoa:

- Rinse one cup of quinoa under cold water.

- In a saucepan, combine quinoa and 2 cups water. Bring to a boil, then decrease heat, cover, and cook for 15-20 minutes, or until the water is absorbed. Fluff with a fork.

For the Grilled Shrimp:

- In a bowl, toss shrimp with 2 tablespoons of olive oil, salt, and pepper. Preheat the grill or grill pan to medium-high heat.

- Grill shrimp for 2-3 minutes per side, until opaque and cooked through.

For the Salad:

- In a large bowl, combine cooked quinoa, grilled shrimp, cherry tomatoes, and diced avocados. In a separate small bowl, whisk together 1/4 cup olive oil, balsamic vinegar, Dijon mustard, salt, and pepper.

- Drizzle the dressing over the salad and gently toss to mix.
- Garnish with fresh parsley.

Nutritional Value (per serving):

- Calories: Approximately 450
- Protein: 25g
- Carbohydrates: 35g
- Fat: 25g
- Fiber: 8g

Cooking Time:

Quinoa: 15-20 minutes

Shrimp: 6-8 minutes

8. Spinach and Feta Stuffed Chicken Breast with Mashed Cauliflower

Ingredients:

- 4 boneless, skinless chicken breasts

- 2 cups fresh spinach, chopped

- cup feta cheese, crumbled

- cloves garlic, minced

- 1 tablespoon olive oil

- Salt and pepper to taste

- Mashed Cauliflower:

- large head cauliflower, chopped

- tablespoons butter

- 1/4 cup heavy cream Salt and pepper to taste

Preparation:

1. Preheat the oven to 375°F (190°C).

2. In a skillet, sauté chopped spinach and minced garlic in olive oil until spinach wilts. Remove from heat and add crumbled feta.

3. Slice a pocket into each chicken breast. Stuff each with the spinach and feta mixture.

4. Season chicken breasts with salt and pepper. Place them in a baking dish.

5. Bake in the preheated oven for 25-30 minutes, or until the chicken is thoroughly done.

For Mashed Cauliflower:

- Steam or boil cauliflower until tender.

- In a food processor, combine cooked cauliflower, butter, and heavy cream. Blend until smooth.

- Season with salt and pepper to taste.

Nutritional Value (per serving):

- Calories: Approximately 400

- Protein: 35g

- Fat: 22g

- Carbohydrates: 15g

- Fiber: 5g

Cooking Time: 45-60 minutes (including prep)

9. Vegetable and Lentil Stew with Whole Grain Bread

Ingredients:

For the Stew:

- cup dry green or brown lentils

- tablespoons olive oil

- onion, diced

- carrots, chopped

- celery stalks, sliced

- cloves garlic, minced

- 1 teaspoon cumin

89

- 1 teaspoon smoked paprika

- 1 can (14 oz) diced tomatoes

- 4 cups vegetable broth

- 2 cups water

- Salt and pepper to taste 2 cups chopped kale or spinach

For the Whole Grain Bread:

- 2 cups whole wheat flour

- 1 cup all-purpose flour

- 1 packet (2 1/4 teaspoons) active dry yeast

- 1 teaspoon salt

- 1 tablespoon honey 1 1/4 cups warm water

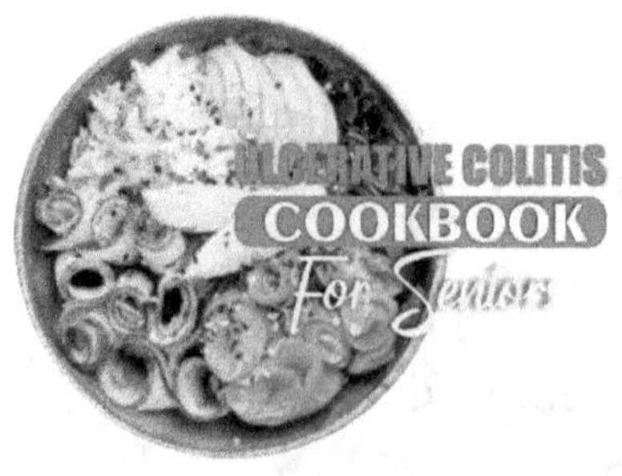

Preparation:

Stew:

1. Rinse the lentils in cool water and leave aside.

2. In a big pot, heat olive oil over medium heat.

3. Add onions, carrots, celery, and garlic; sauté until softened.

4. Add cumin and smoked paprika; stir to coat vegetables.

5. Pour in diced tomatoes, vegetable broth, water, and lentils. Season with salt and pepper. Bring to a boil, then reduce the heat and simmer for 25-30 minutes, or until the lentils are cooked.

6. Add chopped kale or spinach, cook for an additional 5 minutes until greens are wilted.

Nutritional Value:

This stew is rich in fiber, protein, and various vitamins. Approximately 300 calories per serving.

Whole Grain Bread:

1. In a bowl, combine whole wheat flour, all-purpose flour, yeast, and salt.

2. Add honey to warm water, then pour it into the flour mixture. Knead until you have a smooth dough.

3. Let the dough rise in a covered bowl for about 1 hour or until doubled in size.

4. Preheat the oven to 375°F (190°C). Shape the dough and place it in a greased loaf pan.

5. Bake for 30-35 minutes or until the bread sounds hollow when tapped.

Nutritional Value:

• The whole grain bread provides complex carbohydrates, fiber, and essential nutrients.

Cooking Time:

Stew: Approximately 35-40 minutes

Bread: Approximately 30-35 minutes

10. Roasted Turkey Breast with Butternut Squash Mash and Sauteed Kale

Ingredients:

Roasted Turkey Breast:

- turkey breast (about 2.5 lbs)
- tablespoons olive oil
- 1 teaspoon salt
- 1/2 teaspoon black pepper
- 1 teaspoon dried thyme Butternut

Squash Mash:

- medium-sized butternut squash, peeled and diced
- tablespoons butter
- 1/4 cup milk
- Salt and pepper to taste

Sauteed Kale:

- bunch kale, stems removed, leaves cut.
- tablespoons olive oil

- 2 cloves garlic, minced Salt and pepper to taste

Preparation:

Roasted Turkey Breast:

1. Preheat oven to 375°F (190°C).

2. Rub the turkey breast with olive oil, salt, pepper, and dried thyme.

3. Place the turkey breast on a roasting pan and roast for approximately 1.5 hours or until the internal temperature reaches 165°F (74°C).

Butternut Squash Mash:

- Boil the diced butternut squash until tender, then drain.

- Mash the squash with butter, milk, salt, and pepper until smooth.

Sauteed Kale:

- In a medium-size skillet, heat the olive oil.

- Saute minced garlic until fragrant, then add chopped kale. Cook kale until wilted, season with salt and pepper.

Nutritional Value:

- Roasted Turkey Breast (per serving):

- Calories: ~250

- Protein: ~30g

- Fat: ~12g

- Carbohydrates: ~2g

Butternut Squash Mash (per serving):

- Calories: ~120

- Protein: ~2g

- Fat: ~6g

- Carbohydrates: ~20g Sauteed Kale (per serving):

- Calories: ~50

- Protein: ~2g

- Fat: ~4g

- Carbohydrates: ~6g

Cooking Time:

Roasted Turkey Breast: Approximately 1.5 hours

Butternut Squash Mash: 20-25 minutes

Sauteed Kale: 8-10 minutes

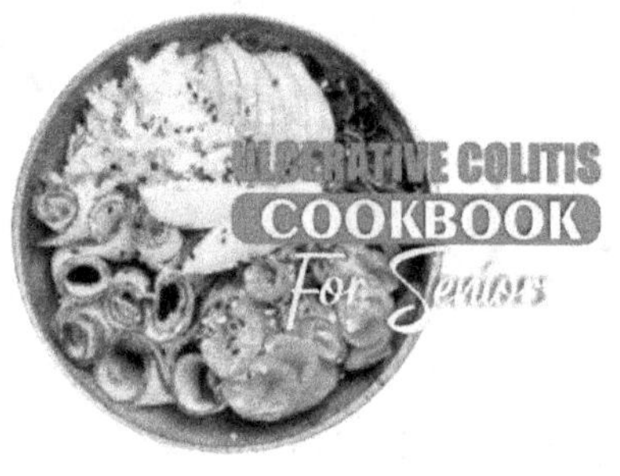

The Paperback Of This Version Has A Free 14 Weeks Meal Planner

MY WEEKLY MEAL PLANNER

Date

	Breakfast	Lunch	Dinner
MON			
TUE			
WED			
THU			
FRI			
SAT			
SUN			

SHOPPING LIST:

To Do List

NOTES AND TIPS

Day 1:

- Breakfast: Oatmeal with mashed banana and ground flaxseeds.
- Lunch: Grilled chicken with steamed carrots and mashed sweet potatoes.
- Dinner: Baked Salmon with Quinoa and Steamed Vegetables.

Day 2:

- Breakfast: Scrambled eggs with spinach and a side of plain yogurt.
- Lunch: Baked salmon with quinoa and roasted zucchini.
- Dinner: Mashed Sweet Potatoes with Grilled Chicken and Green Beans.

Day 3:

- Breakfast: Brown Rice Porridge with Cooked Apples and Honey.
- Lunch: Turkey and vegetable stir-fry with brown rice.
- Dinner: Turkey and Vegetable Stir-Fry with Brown Rice.

Day 4:

- Breakfast: Quinoa and Vegetable Stir-Fry with Soft-Cooked Eggs.
- Lunch: Spinach and feta omelette with a side of roasted bell peppers.
- Dinner: Grilled Tilapia with Lemon Herb Quinoa and Roasted Zucchini.

Day 5:

- Breakfast: Greek yogurt parfait with low-acid fruits like berries and kiwi.
- Lunch: Lentil soup with whole-grain toast.
- Dinner: Chicken and Rice Soup with Carrots and Spinach.

Day 6:

- Breakfast: Smoothie made with ripe banana, almond milk, and nut butter.
- Lunch: Grilled shrimp salad with mixed greens and a light vinaigrette.
- Dinner: Baked Cod with Cilantro Lime Rice and Steamed Asparagus.

Day 7:

- Breakfast: Baked sweet potatoes with a dollop of plain yogurt and chives.

- Lunch: Baked cod with sautéed spinach and quinoa.
- Dinner: Quinoa Salad with Grilled Shrimp, Cherry Tomatoes, and Avocado.

Day 8:

- Breakfast: Cottage cheese with sliced peaches and a handful of walnuts.
- Lunch: Turkey and vegetable wrap with a gluten-free tortilla.
- Dinner: Spinach and Feta Stuffed Chicken Breast with Mashed Cauliflower.

Day 9:

- Breakfast: Buckwheat pancakes with pureed berries as a topping.
- Lunch: Mashed butternut squash with roasted chicken breast.

- Dinner: Vegetable and Lentil Stew with Whole Grain Bread.

Day 10:

- Breakfast: Soft-boiled eggs with steamed spinach and a slice of whole-grain toast.
- Lunch: Quinoa and roasted vegetable bowl with a touch of olive oil.
- Dinner: Roasted Turkey Breast with Butternut Squash Mash and Sauteed Kale.

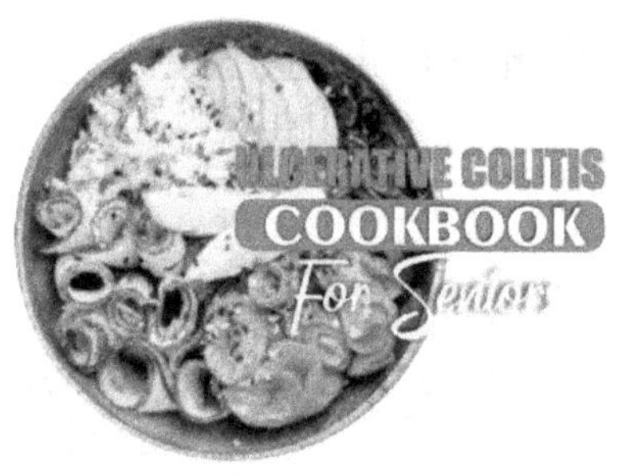

Day 11:

- Breakfast: Oatmeal with mashed banana and a sprinkle of ground flaxseeds.
- Lunch: Grilled chicken with steamed carrots and mashed sweet potatoes.
- Dinner: Baked Salmon with Quinoa and Steamed Vegetables.

Day 12:

- Breakfast: Scrambled eggs with spinach and a side of plain yogurt.
- Lunch: Baked salmon with quinoa and roasted zucchini.
- Dinner: Mashed Sweet Potatoes with Grilled Chicken and Green Beans.

Day 13:

- Breakfast: Brown Rice Porridge with Cooked Apples and Honey.

- Lunch: Turkey and vegetable stir-fry with brown rice.

- Dinner: Turkey and Vegetable Stir-Fry with Brown Rice.

Day 14:

- Breakfast: Quinoa and Vegetable Stir-Fry with Soft-Cooked Eggs.

- Lunch: Spinach and feta omelette with a side of roasted bell peppers.

- Dinner: Grilled Tilapia with Lemon Herb Quinoa and Roasted Zucchini.

Day 15:

- Breakfast: Greek yogurt parfait with low-acid fruits like berries and kiwi.
- Lunch: Lentil soup with whole-grain toast.
- Dinner: Chicken and Rice Soup with Carrots and Spinach.

Day 16:

- Breakfast: Smoothie made with ripe banana, almond milk, and a spoonful of nut butter.
- Lunch: Grilled shrimp salad with mixed greens and a light vinaigrette.
- Dinner: Baked Cod with Cilantro Lime Rice and Steamed Asparagus.

Day 17:

- Breakfast: Baked sweet potatoes with a dollop of plain yogurt and chives.
- Lunch: Baked cod with sautéed spinach and quinoa.
- Dinner: Quinoa Salad with Grilled Shrimp, Cherry Tomatoes, and Avocado.

Day 18:

- Breakfast: Cottage cheese with sliced peaches and a handful of walnuts.
- Lunch: Turkey and vegetable wrap with a gluten-free tortilla.
- Dinner: Spinach and Feta Stuffed Chicken Breast with Mashed Cauliflower.

Day 19:

- Breakfast: Buckwheat pancakes with pureed berries as a topping.

- Lunch: Mashed butternut squash with roasted chicken breast.

- Dinner: Vegetable and Lentil Stew with Whole Grain Bread.

Day 20:

- Breakfast: Soft-boiled eggs with steamed spinach and a slice of whole-grain toast.

- Lunch: Quinoa and roasted vegetable bowl with a touch of olive oil.

- Dinner: Roasted Turkey Breast with Butternut Squash Mash and Sauteed Kale.

Day 21:

- Breakfast: Oatmeal with mashed banana and a sprinkle of ground flaxseeds.

- Lunch: Grilled chicken with steamed carrots and mashed sweet potatoes.

- Dinner: Baked Salmon with Quinoa and Steamed Vegetables.

Day 22:

- Breakfast: Scrambled eggs with spinach and a side of plain yogurt.

- Lunch: Baked salmon with quinoa and roasted zucchini.

- Dinner: Mashed Sweet Potatoes with Grilled Chicken and Green Beans.

Day 23:

- Breakfast: Brown Rice Porridge with Cooked Apples and Honey.

- Lunch: Turkey and vegetable stir-fry with brown rice.

- Dinner: Turkey and Vegetable Stir-Fry with Brown Rice.

Day 24:

- Breakfast: Quinoa and Vegetable Stir-Fry with Soft-Cooked Eggs.

- Lunch: Spinach and feta omelette with a side of roasted bell peppers.

- Dinner: Grilled Tilapia with Lemon Herb Quinoa and Roasted Zucchini.

Day 25:

- Breakfast: Greek yogurt parfait with low-acid fruits like berries and kiwi.
- Lunch: Lentil soup with whole-grain toast.
- Dinner: Chicken and Rice Soup with Carrots and Spinach.

Day 26:

- Breakfast: Smoothie made with ripe banana, almond milk, and a spoonful of nut butter.
- Lunch: Grilled shrimp salad with mixed greens and a light vinaigrette.
- Dinner: Baked Cod with Cilantro Lime Rice and Steamed Asparagus.

Day 27:

- Breakfast: Baked sweet potatoes with a dollop of plain yogurt and chives.
- Lunch: Baked cod with sautéed spinach and quinoa.
- Dinner: Quinoa Salad with Grilled Shrimp, Cherry Tomatoes, and Avocado.

Day 28:

- Breakfast: Cottage cheese with sliced peaches and a handful of walnuts.
- Lunch: Turkey and vegetable wrap with a gluten-free tortilla.
- Dinner: Spinach and Feta Stuffed Chicken Breast with Mashed Cauliflower.

Day 29:

- Breakfast: Buckwheat pancakes with pureed berries as a topping.

- Lunch: Mashed butternut squash with roasted chicken breast.

- Dinner: Vegetable and Lentil Stew with Whole Grain Bread.

Day 30:

- Breakfast: Soft-boiled eggs with steamed spinach and a slice of whole-grain toast.

- Lunch: Quinoa and roasted vegetable bowl with a touch of olive oil.

- Dinner: Roasted Turkey Breast with Butternut Squash Mash and Sauteed Kale.

Congratulations on completing the 30-day meal plan! Feel free to continue incorporating these recipes or explore new ones to maintain a diverse and balanced diet. Enjoy the journey of delicious and nutritious meals!

Finally, this Ulcerative Colitis Cookbook for Seniors is an invaluable resource, providing not just delicious meals but also specialized dietary advice to help manage and reduce the symptoms of this condition. By emphasizing nutrient-dense products and meeting dietary limitations, the cookbook offers seniors a practical and entertaining method to improve their digestive health.

The varied selection of dishes offers a well-balanced and tasty approach to meals, creating a positive relationship with food while meeting the special demands of ulcerative colitis patients. Incorporating this cookbook into daily life not only promotes physical well-being, but also enables seniors to take charge of their health through attentive and joyful eating practices.

As you embark on this gastronomic journey, keep in mind that adopting and adapting to this diet is an effective form of self-care. The carefully chosen meals are more than just nutritious; they lead to a revitalized sense of vitality and resilience. Accept this opportunity to emphasize your well-being, viewing each meal as a step toward a happier and more fulfilled existence. Your devotion to this particular diet is more than just a regimen; it is a celebration of your dedication to a healthy and prosperous future.

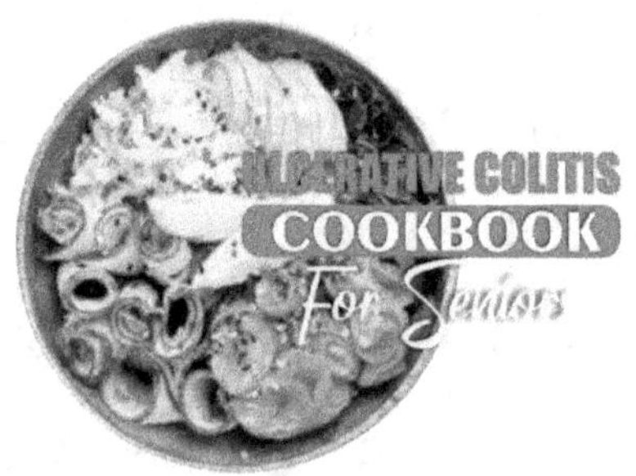

MY WEEKLY MEAL PLANNER

Date

	Breakfast	Lunch	Dinner
MON			
TUE			
WED			
THU			
FRI			
SAT			
SUN			

SHOPPING LIST:

TO DO LIST

NOTES
AND TIPS

MY WEEKLY MEAL PLANNER

Date

	Breakfast	Lunch	Dinner
Mon			
Tue			
Wed			
Thu			
Fri			
Sat			
Sun			

SHOPPING LIST:

- • . . . .
- • . . . .
- • . . . .
- • . . . .

To Do List

. . . .
. . . .
. . . .
. . . .

Notes
And Tips

MY WEEKLY MEAL PLANNER

Date

	Breakfast	Lunch	Dinner
MON			
TUE			
WED			
THU			
FRI			
SAT			
SUN			

SHOPPING LIST:

To Do List

NOTES AND TIPS

MY WEEKLY MEAL PLANNER

Date

	Breakfast	Lunch	Dinner
MON			
TUE			
WED			
THU			
FRI			
SAT			
SUN			

SHOPPING LIST:

TO DO LIST

NOTES
AND TIPS

MY WEEKLY MEAL PLANNER

Date

	Breakfast	Lunch	Dinner
MON			
TUE			
WED			
THU			
FRI			
SAT			
SUN			

SHOPPING LIST:

To Do List

-
-
-
-

NOTES
AND TIPS

MY WEEKLY MEAL PLANNER

Date

	Breakfast	Lunch	Dinner
MON			
TUE			
WED			
THU			
FRI			
SAT			
SUN			

SHOPPING LIST:

To Do List

NOTES AND TIPS

MY WEEKLY MEAL PLANNER

Date

	Breakfast	Lunch	Dinner
MON			
TUE			
WED			
THU			
FRI			
SAT			
SUN			

SHOPPING LIST:

To Do List

- ....
- ....
- ....
- ....

NOTES
AND TIPS

MY WEEKLY MEAL PLANNER

Date

	Breakfast	Lunch	Dinner
Mon			
Tue			
Wed			
Thu			
Fri			
Sat			
Sun			

SHOPPING LIST:

To Do List

- ....
- ....
- ....
- ....

Notes And Tips

MY WEEKLY MEAL PLANNER

Date

	Breakfast	Lunch	Dinner
MON			
TUE			
WED			
THU			
FRI			
SAT			
SUN			

SHOPPING LIST:

To Do List

NOTES
AND TIPS

MY WEEKLY MEAL PLANNER

Date

	Breakfast	Lunch	Dinner
MON			
TUE			
WED			
THU			
FRI			
SAT			
SUN			

SHOPPING LIST:

TO DO LIST

- ● . . . .
- ● . . . .
- ● . . . .
- ● . . . .

NOTES AND TIPS

MY WEEKLY MEAL PLANNER

Date

	Breakfast	Lunch	Dinner
MON			
TUE			
WED			
THU			
FRI			
SAT			
SUN			

SHOPPING LIST:

-
-
-
-

TO DO LIST

NOTES AND TIPS

MY WEEKLY MEAL PLANNER

Date

	Breakfast	Lunch	Dinner
MON			
TUE			
WED			
THU			
FRI			
SAT			
SUN			

SHOPPING LIST:

- ●
- ●
- ●
- ●

TO DO LIST

NOTES AND TIPS

MY WEEKLY MEAL PLANNER

Date

	Breakfast	Lunch	Dinner
MON			
TUE			
WED			
THU			
FRI			
SAT			
SUN			

SHOPPING LIST:

TO DO LIST

-
-
-
-

NOTES AND TIPS

MY WEEKLY MEAL PLANNER

Date

	Breakfast	Lunch	Dinner
MON			
TUE			
WED			
THU			
FRI			
SAT			
SUN			

SHOPPING LIST:

TO DO LIST

NOTES
AND TIPS